THE ACT OF CONSTANT DROWNING

A Journey Through the Waves of Physical and Mental Health

Iona Stuart

The Act of Constant Drowning

ISBN: 978-1-7178-4995-3

The author may be contacted at:
ionamstuart@gmail.com

"Remember about the shadow of past knowledge. Write about your own experience. By that experience, someone else may be a bit richer some day."
– Sylvia Plath

CONTENTS

CHAPTER #1

Introduction

"God, how I ricochet between certainties and doubts."
– Sylvia Plath

Have you ever noticed that no one tells you what it's like to be a person? I mean, one day each of us is just born out of nowhere, and suddenly the universe turns around and says, "You are now a human. Good luck." And when you think about what that means, it's actually kind of terrifying.

Then, as we get older, our worlds begin to shift and grow. Everything we encounter shapes a part of who we become—the others around us, the things that we do, and the choices that we make all have a considerable impact on how we develop as human beings. I find all of that to be somewhat mind-boggling, and half the time, I wish I could go back to the universe and ask for the details of its returns policy.

One of the scary things about being a writer, doing the things that I do, and making some of the choices I have made, is the fact that it really does open up everything for the world to see. It's like putting your soul on show and waiting for the backlash.

One of the main concerns I had about even writing this in the first place was the response I might receive from others.

My number one thought when I began this journey was, "What will my family think?" That was the very first thing to pop into my head. I think this is because, although they are the most supportive people I have in my life, I have a tendency to occasionally disappear off the face of the Earth, and so they don't all know everything that this book is going to address. The other thing about my family is that it's quite large and amazingly complicated, and due to that, I'm pretty sure everyone knows slightly different aspects of my life: those to whom I am closest obviously see a lot more than those with whom I do not have so much contact.

The other group of people to niggle at the back of my brain when writing this was my friends. I did discuss this project with a few of my friends before I started writing, and even used them as an opinion poll for the title of this book—I gave them my three choices and made a tally system based on the ranking they provided (thanks, guys!). Yet, looking at the connections I have on social media, I had this horrible wave of anxiety when I imagined them reading the final product. But the people I actually talked to about it were very supportive, and my best friend was extremely helpful, as she always is.

Another concern that made me hesitant when it came to writing this was the fear of coming across as self-obsessed. When the very idea for this project first came to mind, the automatic internal thought reaction was, "But who wants to read about your life? What makes you so special that you think people would be even remotely interested?"

Those thoughts were particularly daunting, because I couldn't come up with an answer.

In response to all of the concerns and fears regarding writing this book, I guess the obvious thing would be quite simply not to do it, right? If writing openly about aspects of your life and publishing those things in a book or posting about them on a public platform makes you uncomfortable, then you don't have to do it.

But, here's the thing, I am the kind of person who is always fascinated by reading about the lives of others. If I see even the slightest thing posted on social media or something that's being hinted at on a TV show, then I want to know the whole story. So, in that sense, I feel it would be very hypocritical of me to want to know everything about everyone else, and yet not allow anyone to know anything about me.

Even in writing that last sentence, the fear of coming across as self-obsessed started knocking at my door. But (after many hours spent in agonizing contemplation) I have come to the conclusion that these thoughts are something that I just have to accept, and then move on. This is because people do often ask me questions—whether the questions are actually about me, or just about my knowledge or experience in regards to some of the physical or mental health conditions I deal with—and if I stayed silent every time, due to feelings of insecurity, then these questions would remain unanswered. I realized that it would be far more helpful to people if I had everything written down in one place, rather than having a thousand different conversations with a thousand different faces, each discussing slightly different points because I can never quite remember all the relevant things at any one given moment in time.

I tend to be interested in the lives of others because I'm always intrigued to see what I can learn from them. I always want to know how another person's diagnosis story went; how that person deals with their depression or manages their MS relapses; I want to know if other people with epilepsy have had seizures at concerts, and what they did to deal with this situation. I have so many questions that pop up all the time in regards to so many things, be them travel, nutrition, social circumstances, dating, embarrassing moments, etc. And I don't want to read a page in a medical journal, or be overloaded with technical hospital jargon—I want to read stories about real people, who have lived real lives and have learned what works for them.

For example, I follow quite a few body positivity activists on various social media platforms, who share not only a lot of personal pictures but also a lot of personal information about themselves online. I am one of the many people in the world who is very thankful for this. In witnessing their life stories as they unfold and seeing all the things they have overcome, it gives me a boost in my own self-confidence, and helps make me believe that I, too, can overcome the challenges in my life. Especially those that directly relate to mental health and issues with my body image.

So, in writing this, I am really hoping that I can do my part to answer some of the questions that other people out there may have. I want to help by contributing my knowledge and experiences to the community of others who are doing the same, because sharing what we know with the aim of aiding one another is vital to how we all grow and develop as human beings. As I said, I know there are people who do have questions—not only have I met them, but I'm one of them! Also, it really means a lot to me to write about these particular areas, because it would make me so happy to think that maybe (even if only a little bit) this book might help spread some awareness of the topics discussed.

So, let us begin.

CHAPTER #2

Many Scars

"I want to live and feel all the shades, tones and variations of mental and physical experience possible in life. And I am horribly limited."
– Sylvia Plath

W henever I talk to anyone about my life—or even just think to myself about my life—it seems that everything began when I was 14 years old. I believe that this is for a number of reasons, the primary being that I really don't remember very much at all before this age.

Usually, when I explain this to people, I tend to get one of two reactions: either the other person understands entirely and can relate on a personal level to this inability to remember being a kid, or they furrow their brow and question how many times I've hit my head—spoiler alert, the answer to that question is 'a lot!'

To be perfectly honest, although 14 has become my go-to

age, I don't actually remember all that much in the few years that followed. I often joke that every year I live is another year I forget from the past; as if my active memory is a roll of film that keeps on running, but the slides at the beginning keep falling into direct sunlight.

However, aside from the fact that I have the memory of a goldfish, the other main reason why 14 is the age at which my life seemingly began is that this was the age when I was diagnosed with multiple sclerosis.

For anyone who doesn't know, multiple sclerosis (MS) is a condition that affects the central nervous system (CNS). In our bodies, we have this stuff called myelin, which covers the nerve fibers in the CNS. With MS, a person's immune system attacks this myelin sheath, which results in scars or lesions. These lesions interrupt the messages that travel through the nerve fibers, and basically result in things not working so well.

For example, imagine a cellphone charger—you have a bunch of copper wires wrapped in insulation, which carry the current from the power source to your phone. Now, imagine that this insulation becomes damaged—maybe from wear and tear due to how many times you shove it in your bag, or perhaps your cat thought it would be fun to use it as a chew toy—and you find that your charger doesn't work properly anymore. Maybe it takes forever to charge your phone, or the charge jumps in and out while it's plugged in, deciding that sometimes it's going to play ball, and other times it's not.

That's pretty much what happens in MS.

Sometimes, it causes a delay in when signals from the brain are trying to reach certain parts of the body. During some of my relapses, I have to use dictation to write things, because I can't use a keyboard properly (literally, this is a writer's worst nightmare!). This is because although I can still use my fingers, the signals between my brain and my hands become so delayed that I completely lack the dexterity to type.

Other times, it causes a delay in when signals from certain parts of the body are trying to reach the brain. For me, the biggest issue in this department is knowing when I need to pee. The delay in my brain being informed of this information has not ended well on several occasions. Trust me.

The odd thing about my MS diagnosis is that I don't remember what a lot of my initial symptoms were, or how they led me to where they did. The thing I remember most about this period in my life is the fact that I used to get headaches all the time. And I mean *all* the time. Sometimes I would have a single headache that lasted up to 50 days. There are marriages that don't last this long.

At first, I was told that I was experiencing migraines, and was prescribed medication for that. I don't remember a lot about how this came about, or how helpful any of the information I was given at this time actually was, but I do vaguely recall that this drug made me feel like a zombie. So, I stopped taking it. However, over the following years, my random headaches gradually became less frequent, and although I still get headaches quite often, I tend to be able to pinpoint a reason for them these days—seizure hangovers, hitting my head off various surfaces, stress, eyestrain… that sort of thing.

I also developed an issue with my somatosensory system. Hot things were cold, cold things were hot, and you could probably kick me in the shins without me noticing. In fact, there was one day when I was in high school and sitting at a particular desk that was shoved into the corner of the room, next to a radiator. It turned out that my arm was resting against this radiator for the full hour of lesson time, and it wasn't until after class that I noticed the tiger stripe burns on my arm from where it had been touching the heater. And when I say burns, I mean *burns*. They even blistered. But I hadn't recognized that my arm had been leaning against something that was hot.

Another thing I sort of remember is that I was constantly dizzy, and this is something that has never changed. Three years later, at the age of 17, I was prescribed drugs for the purpose of making me feel less like my world was spinning, and I continue to take medication for this today. I'm still not sure what causes this exactly, but the drugs work, so I can't really complain.

One thing I definitely remember, however, is that it was amazingly difficult trying to get answers from doctors. I feel like this is something to which a lot of people can relate. It is so frustrating when you know that your body is not functioning the way it should be, and yet every time you go to a doctor, it almost turns into an argument.

There is a specific memory about this that sticks in my mind, possibly due to how ridiculous the whole appointment turned out to be. Now, let me start by saying that I am a self-confessed stress head; the majority of things in the world make me stressed—in fact, I actually have a list that I call, 'Simple Things, Which Cause Me Undue Stress'—and it has certainly caused problems in my life, some of which have manifested physically. However, when going to a doctor in regards to not being able to tell whether or not the object I am touching is going to burn me, I did not expect the response to be, "It's probably just stress."

What was the advice I was given? To listen to a whale noises tape. Seriously.

I also had a doctor who suggested that every one of my health concerns was caused by caffeine intolerance, and all I had to do to be cured was stop drinking cola. Okay, so it did turn out that I have a sensitivity to caffeine, and so have not knowingly consumed any (I was only recently informed that chocolate contains caffeine, oops) for about three years now—but still!

Eventually, I fell into the sightline of doctors who were a bit more helpful, and after some fun tests—including a lumbar puncture, an electrocution game that involved sending currents between my feet and my head, and numerous MRI scans—I was diagnosed with multiple sclerosis.

When I was first diagnosed, I was put on a type of medication that I had to self-inject three times a week. It's pretty safe to say that I am not a person who is scared of needles (as anyone may have guessed from the number of body piercings and tattoos that I have), and I think one of the main reasons for this is because I got used to shoving them into my subcutaneous tissue on a regular basis.

I would inject on Mondays, Wednesdays, and Fridays, rotating between both of my thighs and my abdomen. The reason the injection site had to be rotated was due to a side effect that caused damage to the surrounding tissue and resulted in these painful hard lumps just beneath the skin.

However, although I wasn't against having to take the injections, I wasn't exactly a fan either and did have a tendency to screw it up sometimes. I was especially good at hitting minor veins, which could be kind of painful and often caused bruises and bleeding. I also strongly advise against any self-injecting while intoxicated, because I actually did that quite a lot in my younger teenage years and I can assure you that it never ends well.

Along with all the injections came a new addition to my room—Fred the Friendly Sharps Box. Now, I have absolutely no idea why I felt the need to name my sharps box Fred, but I stuck a label on him and everything. He was my little orange friend who sat atop my chest of drawers, and happily ate all of my used syringes. He also helpfully hid the gas-sterilized hollow needles I used to use to give myself new body piercings. Thanks, Fred: I

17

could never have pierced my own navel at 15 without you.

The most irritating thing that I found with having to take a medication that required injection was what to do when traveling, especially when said medication had to be kept at certain temperatures. In general, when traveling around the civilized world, this was not so much of an issue. But when you're shipped off to school camp and spend a week moving between campsites and hostels in the middle of nowhere, it can be super annoying.

Something else that I found sort of odd was the interest that others had in watching me inject. I had a few friends who asked to watch, which I could understand was probably due to a mixture of sheer curiosity and wanting to see if someone as clumsy as I could really shove a syringe in my thigh correctly. But I also had a few not-friends who asked to watch—school acquaintances who were seemingly intrigued by the injection process. Either that or they just had some really strange kinks.

Another thing that really characterized these early years of my MS diagnosis was my lack of coordination and inability to move quickly. At certain points, I literally had to have another person fasten the buttons on my blouse or help me tie my shoes, because my fingers did not want to play those games. I also like to think back and remember myself as quite a fast sprinter (but maybe I made that up inside my head, I'm not entirely sure), and during these years surrounding my diagnosis, I was utterly unable to run. What I think is so weird about this is that, as far as

I'm aware, my walking wasn't really affected so much at this point in time (or at least not to the extent that I have since experienced), so how come my running was?

I'm pretty sure this was something to do with the signals between my brain and my legs being delayed. The messages still got through, hence how I was able to walk, but the speed required for running was just not feasible. And so, instead of taking off quickly when my brain said, "Run!" I ended up just falling over after about two or three strides. This was something that other students at my high school found to be highly amusing, and there may or may not still be a video or two of me floating around the internet somewhere.

My diagnosis was one of Relapse-Remitting MS (RRMS), and I spent the majority of the following years in a state of remission. As the years progressed, I was lucky enough not to experience many issues related to this aspect of my health and was pretty much able to live as if this thing did not exist in my life. From time to time, I still had some problems concerning coordination, and my ability to distinguish between hot and cold could occasionally be a bit questionable. However, this did not limit me at all, and I was able to lead a perfectly 'normal' life.

Then, at the age of 16, I moved to boarding school in England. (*Pop quiz!* How many movies can you think of that begin with that cliché?) Just before I moved, my medication was switched from the injections I had been taking, to a capsule drug. This made me very happy! Although I had never really hated taking the injections, I did find them to be somewhat inconvenient and was definitely anxious about the idea of moving into a boarding house carrying a bunch of syringes that required refrigeration, and a sharps box (no matter how friendly).

I think some people cringe slightly when they hear the words 'boarding school,' and imagine scenes from Dickens' *A Christmas Carol*. But I can honestly say that boarding school was the best thing that ever happened to me. I grew so much as a person in those two years than I had in the four years previous that I'd spent at my first high school.

While staying in England, I became very active, both physically and socially. I went to the onsite gym maybe five or six times a week; I walked around the York city walls on the weekends; and I attended a few evening club activities, like badminton. I also did a lot of baking, and I mean *a lot* of baking. I baked for clubs, charity events, English class cake days, and also just for fun.

And during this time, which turned out to be massively life changing, I was incredibly grateful that this condition did not hold me back from getting out there and living. This long period of remission was essentially like getting to be on break from having MS for a few years.

But the thing about having a condition like this is that one can get far too comfortable during remission, and then when relapse comes back around, it feels sort of like a slap in the face. Or at least this is what it was like for me. While in the midst of my worst relapses, I was amazed at just how much I couldn't do—especially since the changes seemed to take place practically overnight. It's like, I would go to bed one evening, and the next morning, I'd wake up unable to move properly.

During these types of full-blown relapse, the main issue I have these days is that I can't really walk very well. I become super uncoordinated, experience numbness that spans from the waist down (or sometimes it even starts up at my chest), and some things decide that they're just not going to move at all—toes refuse to wiggle, and legs won't lift. Things like showering and getting dressed suddenly become these massive endeavors.

Lack of dexterity in my hands also means that I can't use a pen, which becomes a problem when asked to fill out a form or sign my name—have you ever noticed how often you need to provide your signature for something? Yeah, it's a pain. And weakness in my arms (coupled with my staggering walking style) makes it impossible for me to cook food, as I can't hold things like pots and pans, am not coordinated enough to navigate an oven without burning myself, and can't carry a plate of food and walk at the same time. Making hot drinks is another no-no. Basically, what this boils down to is that I end up living mainly on toast and apples.

However, I definitely find the worst relapse symptoms to be the tremendously entertaining bathroom troubles. Because I go numb below the waist, when it comes to actions that go on *down there*, all things feel the same. Half the time I don't know when I need to go to the bathroom; and the other half of the time, I know I have to go to the bathroom, but can't. The latter is called urinary retention, and it is really, *really* frustrating. The outcome for not being able to urinate on demand means that the bladder does not get emptied, and so remains nice and full until your brain tells you to do something else, at which point the floodgates suddenly decide to open.

Apparently, the numb half of my body below the waist cannot differentiate between the commands 'walk' and 'pee.' *Well done, body—gold star.*

Altogether, I find that being in MS relapse is very much like being a toddler: I can't walk properly, I can't write letters, going to the bathroom is a skill I don't really have, and I am somewhat unable to perform the most basic tasks of taking care of myself. And I feel like I need a hug. Like, all the time.

As the years pass, and I grow older, I am definitely becoming more aware of the impact that MS can have on my life, especially given the fact that it really can just appear out of nowhere.

I think one of the things about being diagnosed young was that I didn't really have any sense of what it meant for my future. I mean, at the age of 14, I didn't really do much. During these years, being in MS relapse just meant that things at school could be more difficult, and every so often I'd fall off the bus because my legs would buckle at the little steps. But I didn't have to deal with finding and keeping a job; I didn't have to go grocery shopping and cook food for myself; I didn't really have to do anything but go to school, and make sure I finished my homework.

I didn't have to be an adult because I wasn't; and then, suddenly, I was.

The transition to adulthood, for me, meant learning how to be disabled. All of a sudden, this whole world of complications opened up ahead of me, and I had to know how to access the appropriate help and services in order to survive. I was somehow expected to navigate and complete a thousand different forms, all of which made me want to tear my hair out.

There was so much to learn—and I'm nowhere near done trying to figure it all out, especially since I have a tendency to move around—because I had never come across any of this stuff before. I had to research disability payment as I came to terms with the fact that I cannot expect to be able to go out and work all the time, despite my enthusiasm. I also had a whole bunch of fun trying to figure out who I was even supposed to contact in the first place in regards to accessing assistance—and, to be perfectly honest, this still sort of alludes me.

What I ended up doing, was making what I call my 'Disability Life Plan.' This is a plan that I made on my computer, which details all the sorts of practical things I require help with when I'm in relapse. I feel like this is a very useful document to have, as it enables me to get all the stuff I might need to be organized into one place, and means that when the state of my health does take a nosedive, then I'm not left totally stuck and unable to do anything. It also gives me a good basis for knowing what sort of help to look for whenever, and wherever, I relocate.

I started this by noting down all the things that cause me trouble, and the stuff that I can't do. I then added in what support I would need to be able to get certain things done.

For example, I can't always cook when I'm in relapse, so the support that I need to deal with that is a delivery system for groceries and someone who can then come and make food for me. I mean, as much as I'd probably enjoy living on pizza delivery for months at a time, this would probably not be the healthiest decision (and would also be obscenely expensive).

As I said previously, this really was something that I had to learn. I know it may sound strange to suggest 'learning how to be disabled,' but it's true. This is because it's not something that everyone with health conditions just magically knows; you need to have the right information and know where you can access help, and then how to use that information to get everything into place, and it's just not possible to do it all on your own.

Another big part of this process is learning to accept all of these changes and limitations, which can be really fucking hard. I mean, going from being able to do most things, to not (sometimes overnight), is a difficult thing to comprehend. You wake up one morning, and suddenly you're not able to be as independent anymore—even for the most basic, and sometimes embarrassing, of things. And it can be complicated to try and explain to other people (especially people you don't know on a particularly personal level) how last week you were, seemingly, a fully functioning person, and now you can't walk around the grocery store without pissing your pants—both literally and figuratively, depending on how anxious your lack of control may make you feel.

It can result in feeling very trapped in certain situations. I have often sat and wondered, "How am I supposed to detach myself from a toxic environment in order to survive and thrive in my own life when disability makes practical independence a bitch?"

It's at times like this that I'm reminded of the importance of having supportive people in your life, because it can be so emotionally draining to try and do it all on your own, even if you really want to. I am generally quite an independent person, and can certainly be very stubborn when it comes to admitting that I need help. Admitting that you cannot function as a person is a really difficult thing to do, and when you feel like you're giving up your independence, it's not surprising that your mind wants to fight against it. It is not easy.

However, one thing that I have come to realize—and believe me when I say that it took a very long time, and the right people telling me this for me to acknowledge it—is that life really can be made a little bit easier by just asking for help.

CHAPTER #3

Electric Storms

"I am learning how to compromise the wild dream ideals and the necessary realities without such screaming pain."
– Sylvia Plath

I was officially diagnosed with epilepsy about three weeks after my 18th birthday, and I actually recall enough of what happened to tell this story in some detail! Although, in all fairness, I did reread every one of my hospital letters from these two months just before I started writing this chapter, so...

The process of being diagnosed with epilepsy was essentially centered around two specific events—however, as with the MS, there is more of a history behind it than just these particular moments.

The first of these events took place during my 18th birthday celebrations. A few friends and I went out for dinner and drinks in York, and from the pictures that I have of the evening, and the little I do remember, I think we had a pretty good time! The last thing about that night that I specifically recall is ordering pitchers of mojitos for the table, and I think the reason that this sticks in my mind so much is due to the fact that I never got to drink them!

Apparently, what happened next was that I fell off my chair, unconscious, and began convulsing. The next fully formed memory I hold in my brain of that weekend is waking up at about 13:00 the next day in my friend's room, in her bed, and wearing a pair of her pajamas—and thinking, "How the hell did I get here?"

So, how *did* I get there? Well, my magical friends were somehow able to maneuver me into a taxi at some point during my postictal phase (altered state of consciousness following a seizure), and safely escort me back to my friend's house. Her mother then called an ambulance, and some paramedics came and checked me over—this is a part I do not recall—before I was left to rest and sleep it off.

The second of these events took place 19 days later. The day had started out in a way that was, by this point in my life, somewhat normal: I passed out in one of my classes—it was English, by the way, just in case anyone was curious. Following my usual loss of consciousness, I ended up at the school medical center (just like always) and rested there (just like normal). However, what took place on this particular day turned out to be *not* just like normal, and at some point while I was there that afternoon, I had a tonic-clonic seizure.

The nurses at the medical center—who also happen to be some of the most wonderful women in the world—called an ambulance, and I was taken to the local hospital. It was while I was at this hospital that I received my diagnosis: epilepsy secondary to multiple sclerosis.

Although I wasn't diagnosed with epilepsy until I was 18, the length of time I have actually been experiencing seizures is more questionable. This is because a part of the medical issues that began in my younger teenage years included passing out a lot, and no one really knew why.

For a long time, I passed out on a fairly regular basis, and there never seemed to be any sort of identifying link between these occasions. I mean, yes, there were definitely times where my inability to retain consciousness could potentially be blamed on having skipped breakfast, or possible dehydration, or low blood pressure (which is something I do have); however, there were also all the other times when none of these things were relevant, and I still passed out.

The majority of the time, I would just be sitting somewhere, and then—*bam!* Lights out. Hit the deck. I sometimes wish I could have left some sort of marker behind, like maybe a sticker, in all the places I've lost consciousness during my lifetime: it would make one hell of a scavenger hunt.

In my younger teenage years, I also often had sleep paralysis, during which I would be woken up by sounds of screaming, laughter, and rabble that I couldn't quite place. I would be able to see shadows—like demons—on the walls and ceiling, reaching down for me, trying to grab at me and pull me into whatever void they came from. I would be unable to move, then I would feel my body stiffen, feel my lungs clench, hear a rasping squeal as the air was forced through my esophagus, unable to breathe. And then nothing. Sleep paralysis was not fun, and I am so glad that I don't experience this anywhere near as much as I used to.

However, due to this, when I started experiencing what I later went on to learn were nocturnal seizures, I thought that perhaps it was just the sleep paralysis experimenting with new ways of messing with me. But these new events were different, and they would leave me exhausted, sore, and nauseous. I would have a headache that lasted all day, sometimes bites at the back of my tongue or in my cheeks, and one day I awoke having cracked one of my molars. I once sprained my wrist after essentially punching my bedroom wall during one of these events, and often found that things had fallen off the shelf by my bed due to the mini earthquakes that I invoked.

It wasn't actually until I was going over my history with a specialist nurse that we began to realize how much of what I'd previously experienced had most likely been caused by undiagnosed epilepsy. This was put down to the strong possibility that I'd been having secondarily generalized seizures (but without tonic-clonic convulsions), mixed in with other episodes of neurocardiogenic syncope (fainting). Due to the mixture of the two, the fact that I was an adolescent female, and also had generally low blood pressure, things were largely left alone.

Well, you know, until it wasn't possible to leave them alone anymore.

When a person has a seizure, what essentially happens is that there are surges of electrical activity in their brain, and these bursts of activity affect how the brain functions. There is a lot of medical literature out there that likens seizures to electric storms. I really like this analogy, because thinking of the inside of my head as a landscape for electric storms—complete with cracks of thunder and bolts of lightning—makes me feel better about myself. It reminds me of Zeus and makes me feel like epilepsy is more of a secret superpower than a disability.

I realize that I've already used a few 'epilepsy words' in this chapter, the most recurrent being 'tonic-clonic.' This is a type of seizure. There are actually a whole bunch of different types of seizure, but I am not a doctor, so I'm not even going to try to explain them all. The medical powers that be also have this fun tendency to change the names of seizures every so often—just to add to the confusion. However, what I can do is explain what I experience.

The line that crops up in the 'diagnosis' section on all of my medical letters is, 'simple and complex partial seizures, with secondary generalization and tonic-clonic.' So, what does that mean?

Well, partial seizures (also called focal seizures) happen in only one part of the brain.

When I have simple partial seizures, I'm consciously aware

of whatever the seizure is causing, even if I don't always know why. Sometimes these are sensory, and I can smell things that aren't there (usually fish, for some reason), or taste metal. But the taste of metal isn't a taste I have on my tongue, but a taste that I can feel in my nose. It's like some sort of flavor aroma that hangs around my soft palate. If I stop and think it over for long enough, then my brain gets really amazed by the fact that I can smell and taste things that aren't there, and it feels remarkably mind-blowing. So, I try not to think about it too much, for the fear that my head might explode.

The other type of simple partial seizure I experience affects the part of my brain that controls emotion, which has varying results. Sometimes I get a strong sense of either déjà vu or jamais vu, and other times I just laugh or cry hysterically. Both are fun and not fun in about equal measure.

During complex partial seizures, however, I am not consciously aware of what's going on. It's sort of like the world just sticks a pair of 'confusion goggles' over my eyes, and everything suddenly becomes very surreal. I often don't remember what actually occurs during these seizures, but I do have a sort of general sense of things not being right. From what people have told me, what tends to happen is that I'll stop being able to communicate properly, and sort of just sit and stare at things, seemingly analyzing every minute detail of my surroundings, as if seeing everything in the whole world for the very first time. I've also been told that I have a tendency to play with my hands or grind my teeth.

The tonic-clonic (also known as grand mal) part of my diagnosis refers to the type of seizure that people usually think about when they hear the word 'epilepsy.' You know, the unconscious, limbs jerking, eye-rolling type of seizures that they show in the movies. This is a type of generalized seizure, which affects both sides of the brain, and is something that I experience secondary to partial seizures. This means that my seizures start off in one part of the brain (as partial seizures), and if they spread to my whole brain, that then results in generalized seizures.

However, not all generalized seizures present as tonic-clonic, which is one of the main reasons why my history of random unconsciousness was questioned so much after I received my epilepsy diagnosis.

So, I was at boarding school when I was diagnosed with epilepsy. What I find so funny about this is that I think back to the anxiety I had regarding what it might have been like to deal with self-injections while living on a school campus, and all the irritants it could potentially have caused, and then realize that due to my seizures, I ended up being extremely irritating anyway.

As much as I tried to keep a seizure diary (doctors like it when you do this), I still ended up losing track of just how often I had seizures. However, I do have some half-memories of all the things I interrupted during my time at that school, some of which are semi-hilarious—well, in retrospect, anyway.

I certainly disrupted a lot of classes, quite a few school assemblies, and a number of silent Quaker Meetings (I still cringe at that last one). I also had a tendency to make my presence known at some other places on site, from the public platform of the dining hall—I once bruised in the shape of a perfect right angle after falling against the corner of a table—to the privacy of my bedroom—apparently I totally freaked out my roommate when I fell out of bed during a tonic-clonic nocturnal seizure.

However, I think the most hilarious memory I have is definitely coercing a paramedic into helping me escape from the ER (before I'd even been seen by a doctor) so that I could get back to campus on time for Parents' Evening. The best part about this is that I had absolutely no reason for needing to get back—one of the fun parts about being a boarding student is that you don't actually have to take parents to Parents' Evening, you can just go do it by yourself. But I was, in my postictal state, totally sure that this was super important, and that I had to be there. Ultimately, I think all that ended up coming from that decision was me spilling hot tea all over my hands as I vacantly nodded at whatever the teachers were saying, not absorbing a single word. This account sums me up as a person pretty well.

One thing that I was highly aware of at the time, and still think back on very fondly to this day, was the amazing support that I received from the staff at my second high school. The teachers were really great, and not only when I was annoying enough to have seizures during their classes, but also when it came to managing my workload, and helping me make sure that I didn't fall too far behind during the times when I was too brain dead to do anything.

I have already made a brief mention of the wonderful nurses that worked at the school medical center, but they truly were amazing. They were the glue that held me together during the times that were the most difficult and dealt not only with my physical inability to function as a human, but also my numerous emotional breakdowns. They held me up for two years when I felt like crumbling, and I owe a lot of my personal growth to the support they gave me.

I also learned a lot during this time about what I can and cannot expect to be able to do in life. As much as no one really wants to talk about epilepsy as something that places limits on your life, once I knew what I was dealing with, I did have to learn (as I did with the MS) to put certain boundaries in place.

I now think about things more, and try to avoid situations where there is a high risk of triggering a seizure, or where having a seizure would be so dangerous that it's just not worth doing. Some of these things are blatantly obvious, like scuba diving or free-form rock climbing. But others are dangerous in a more subtle sort of way.

One of the main things that I avoid is submerging myself in any body of water. Ever. I don't go swimming, I stay very far away from the ocean, and I do not take baths. Some people may view this fear as somewhat irrational—and I think a part of it possibly is—but in my brain, the risk of physically drowning is not worth it. I mean, my seizures are sub-optimally controlled and still quite frequent, and since I tend to have partial seizures that then progress to generalized seizures, at no point do I have the ability to remove myself from the water.

I also found out through practical experience that concerts are a no-no. This is particularly annoying because I'll see tour dates from my favorite bands, get minorly excited, and then recall what happened the last time I went to a concert, which inevitably leads to some disgruntled groaning.

The last time I went to a concert, it did not end well. My friend and I went to see a gothic metal band, of which I have been a fan since before I can remember (i.e. before the age of 14), and, of course, a large part of their performance included the relentless usage of strobe lighting. Essentially, this led to me crashing through the front barrier between the mosh pit and the stage in the midst of a tonic-clonic seizure. The silver lining, however, was that the lead singer (of whom I am a huge fan) apparently jumped off the stage, after she'd finished the song, to come help! The next thing I vaguely remember is some bouncer carrying me backstage, where I practically dozed off until the end of the show. Once the show was over, the lead singer came back and made sure I was okay and gave me a hug. She was a really nice person; I just wish I remembered more of our encounter.

An interesting thing that I have learned over the course of my epilepsy journey is that, for me, certain frequencies of sound can trigger seizures. This has caused a variety of issues, and once made for a particularly eventful trip to the opera.

Another discovery I had is that fireworks are bad, m'kay? From the Epcot Center to the school Bonfire Night, fireworks and I have had a poor relationship. They may be all the way up in the sky, but they are still very 'flashy flashy,' and my brain cannot deal with that. In fact, I think that because they're up in the sky, it actually makes them worse to deal with; they have the whole canvas of night to illuminate the world above my head with their bedazzling lights.

However, I think that perhaps the hang-up I have that confuses people the most is my dislike of going to the movies. This isn't something that I actively avoid, and I do still go to movie theaters sometimes, but it can take a degree of convincing, and some research into the likelihood of the movie containing flashing images. The reason for this is quite simply because I get nervous if I don't know what extent of flashiness may be involved, and it makes me a little uncomfortable to be in a dark room with a very large screen that I don't have the power turn off if things get bad.

And it's not even just specific flashiness that can cause an issue; I once had a seizure at a screening of *The Jungle Book* because the fast motion in one of the scenes meant that too many inadvertent flickers of different colors entered my brain all at once.

If it wasn't evident by this point in the book, I am the kind of person who likes to make jokes about my epilepsy, because it's just a part of my life, and some of the things that happen as a result can be quite funny. I mean, when I end up throwing a glass of water all down myself due to myoclonic twitching, then it's almost impossible not to laugh. However, as much as I like to try and see the funny side, epilepsy can also have a significant impact on my mental health.

As I mentioned previously, I have quite a track record of disrupting things, and sometimes it just makes me feel like I ruin everything.

Let's take the concert, for example. I later found out what had actually happened was that the house lights came on, and the whole thing was basically put on pause until they got me backstage. I discovered these details by coming across an article about the show online. Not only was this horrendously embarrassing to be told, but I also felt so awful for all the inconvenience this must have caused everyone. I don't know the logistics of any of this, but just imagining the light technicians having to stop the display, the band trying to keep the audience occupied in the unexpected interruption, and the confusion (and possible annoyance) of the people in attendance when everything just suddenly stops, makes me cringe and feel so angry with myself.

Even when I think back to less public moments, like all the times I brought classes to a premature end, it just makes me want to hide. I can't help but think about all the other people's learning experiences that I impacted during this time. I often wonder how anyone ever learned anything when one of their classmates would just hit the deck at any given moment, and stop everything in its tracks.

And then when you multiply this feeling of ruining everything by the number of times I've disrupted other things—including family outings, holiday celebrations, *funeral receptions*, and various types of parties (even my own 18th)—it adds up to a smothering weight of self-loathing.

As well as feeling like I'm a catalyst for ruining everyone's time, epilepsy is also the reason that I have not been able to continue with certain paths in my life. I only survived two months at university before I had to make the decision to drop out due to medical reasons. Because of the frequency of my seizures, and the recovery time involved, I couldn't keep up with the workload, and had very little idea of what was going on most of the time. I also found that I wasn't really able to partake in most of the social aspects of university life, because I was too scared of having seizures out in public, and so I didn't really leave my accommodation. This ultimately led to me sitting in my room drinking wine most of the time.

There was a particularly bad period in regards to my epilepsy when I had about seven months of daily seizure activity. I don't know if it was something to do with the amount of time I spent either unconscious or asleep, but my mind really disconnected from my body during this period. It reached a point where I didn't even really 'feel' the seizures anymore. The weirdness of partial seizures had become my new reality, and the generalized seizures seemed like they were happening to someone else. Then when they switched my meds, my mental health went downhill. One reason for this is that I'd already lost quite a bit of my touch on reality due to my brain physically failing to process the world in the preceding months, but that was then combined with the fact that one of the main side effects of my new medication was an increase in depressive emotion and suicidal thoughts.

Another part of having epilepsy that affects my mental health is the fact that I constantly feel like a burden. I hate the pressure it puts on people to even be around me—my family, my friends, my roommates—because, at the end of the day, they are the ones who are left to deal with it all when I'm incapable of being a person and taking care of myself.

Not every seizure I have is a specifically big deal, and most of the time I just sleep it off, and everything's fine. But there are other occasions when my seizures are somewhat worse, which means that I suddenly become this huge responsibility to the people around me. Sometimes things reach emergency status, and I've woken up more than once in the ICU.

When things like that happen, the feeling of not being capable enough to merely exist as a human being can be overwhelming.

And the frustration of continually ending up in embarrassing situations can really get on top of you and can be very isolating if you cut yourself off from the world in an attempt to try and deal with that. Just like the issues I mentioned in regards to the MS, there can be the same lack of independence that is so highly craved and times when it seems almost impossible to just be a person. I often find that this leads to me feeling very out of control.

However, I do think that feelings of low self-confidence and embarrassment are common in those of us with epilepsy, especially when our seizures are sub-optimally controlled. But what has really helped me the most has been repeating thoughts of self-acceptance over and over again in my mind, mixed in with words of support from those around me. I always try to keep in mind whenever anything happens—even those most embarrassing moments, like disturbing a silent Quaker Meeting—that these events are not my fault. Yes, they can be disruptive, and yes, they can be annoying and embarrassing, but I do not ask for this to be a part of my life, and it is not something that I can control.

This may sound obvious, but I find that just reminding myself that this is not my fault sometimes makes me feel less guilty and less embarrassed. It's acceptance in the form of realizing that this is a part of who I am; sometimes things are better, and sometimes things are worse, but I have to continue anyway.

CHAPTER #4
Clueless Control Freak

"I saw myself sitting in the crotch of this fig tree, starving to death, just because I couldn't make up my mind which of the figs I would choose."
– Sylvia Plath

My issues with food could potentially be traced back to when I was about 14 (there's that age again), simply due to some of the things that I look back on now and am able to think, "Wait a minute, that was not normal, that was not a healthy relationship to have with food." But these issues definitely became more apparent around the age of 16.

This was something that I didn't talk about, or even really recognize, for quite some time. I feared that people would judge me because of my other medical problems and would say that my seizures were worse because of my eating disorder—because I'm not taking care of my body. And now, at this point in my life, I am definitely able to see that. I can recall numerous times when I've woken up in the hospital after seizures, hooked up to IV fluids following the discovery of some electrolyte imbalance or another.

However, as much as there is indeed an argument for how my disordered eating habits affected my epilepsy, there is also the irrefutable fact that my epilepsy had a considerable influence on my disordered eating habits.

This may sound strange, but let me explain. By this point in my life, I had struggled with odd, terrifying, wonderful sensations for years, and I never knew what caused them. No one understood, and I couldn't explain, and I felt like I was going crazy. And, to be perfectly honest, a lot of other people made me feel that way, too.

To some extent, I've always been the kind of person who's susceptible to unhealthy coping mechanisms. I've always had this strange inbuilt need for control and order, and during these years of undiagnosed seizures, and numb body parts that didn't want to respond to my commands, I felt utterly helpless. I had no control over my mind, over my body, over my *life*. There was no structure, no safety net, and no sort of organization to keep my world in line.

But then I discovered that I could control food, I could control what I ate; no one could put food in my mouth but me. It was a way of making my body do what I wanted, setting a goal to work toward, with a plan of how to achieve that goal. It made me feel like I had purpose, and that I was capable of doing something.

The irony in this, of course, is that it doesn't work like that.

There was no control; it was merely an illusion.

What happened instead was that I found myself confined by numbers—the number on the scale, the number on the tape measure, the number of calories in every morsel of anything that may potentially pass my lips. I would set myself these impossible goals, all centered around these numbers—and if I didn't reach the goals? Well, then I would spend hours berating myself, telling myself that I was disgusting, worthless, and would always be a failure. And then I would have to set new and *even stricter* goals, which, in turn, led to the cycle starting all over again. I kept telling myself that *next time* I would be better, *next time* I would succeed, and then I would be in total control.

And that was the illusion. All it ever really did was stop me from participating in things I should have enjoyed, made a lot of situations unnecessarily uncomfortable, and put quite a bit of strain on meaningful relationships with others.

As I said previously, this is another thing that I can now trace back to those early teenage years, which really were oh so much fun. But at the time, I didn't recognize it at all. There was no part of me that thought my relationship with food during these years was unhealthy, and I think that's due to the fact that it wasn't anything to do with the food, but was instead a direct response to how I dealt with everything else that was going on in my life.

During these early years, I didn't count calories, I never weighed myself, I set no plans or goals, and had no obsessive routines—that all came later. However, I did have a weird relationship with food in general, which just happened to manifest in such a way that I didn't even realize it was there.

At this point in my life, I would say that I loved food. I ate almost everything, and thought this was because I enjoyed doing so; but, in reality, when I think back over this time, what I actually did was binge on everything.

Almost every night, I would just sit and eat junk food for hours. I would get off the bus after school and buy bags of candy on the way home, then sit and eat all of it before I started my homework. I would literally unbuckle my school kilt, and just sit in my tights and blouse eating a 200g bar of chocolate, washing it down with about a pint of milk, before I would even think about doing anything else with my life. This was my daily unwind. I ate as a form of comfort. Then, on the weekends, I could easily go through a large multipack bag of crisps, a few bags of popcorn, and possibly a six-pack of beer.

And this was on top of meals.

When I say 'meals,' I guess what I really mean is dinner. I would very rarely eat breakfast, and sometimes when it was brought up to me in my room when I was getting ready for school in the mornings, I would pull bits of it apart and hide other bits, so it looked liked I had eaten. However, when it did come to dinner, I would, once again, eat everything. In fact, not only would I eat dinner, but I also had a tendency to attack any leftovers with a fork straight from the container.

Now, lunch was a little more complicated. It wasn't really

something I ever did, but the reasons why this was the case still elude me. When I first started high school, I developed a refusal to enter the school lunch hall. This was mainly due to the fact that I was not really a fan of being in a loud environment with a lot of other people, and the whole act of queuing to enter the hall, queuing to get the food, and then finding somewhere to sit and eat was so anxiety-provoking that I eventually just refused to do it.

This is actually something that never fully resolved; even years later when I was at boarding school, I still had considerable anxieties about entering the lunch hall and often didn't do it. Even now, when I visit as an Old Scholar and someone suggests meeting over lunch in the hall, my heart still skips a beat. (And, in all honesty, the last time I met with someone this way I just sat at a table and spoke to them as they ate, because I still can't, to this day, deal with the process that is school lunches.)

At some point during my attendance at my first high school, one of my teachers caught on to the fact that I avoided the lunch hall like the plague, and set up this great system where I would, instead of going into the hall, collect school-made packed lunches from reception and eat them elsewhere. This sounded like the perfect solution, and I'm very grateful that was put in place. However, what this led to, ultimately, was me ending up with a locker stashed full of uneaten cheese rolls, which would sit there and decompose for months. I do not know why. I also did not realize this was a problem.

But clearly, it was.

As I mentioned previously, these issues were definitely something that became more apparent when I was 16, at boarding school. I think that this was because, at this point in my life, I was dealing with so many things that I couldn't control in regards to my health (especially epilepsy), and so I clung to the one thing I thought I could control.

This was the age at which I became a slave to the numbers, and the routines, and the rituals that came to define my eating habits. Because I had more independence during this time regarding what and when I ate—as opposed to when I was younger and essentially just waited to be given meals—I felt like I was the captain of my own body, and the feeling of power that gave me was addictive.

One thing of which I wasn't aware at the time, but could see very clearly when reading over my old journal entries, was the strong religious undertone to many of my disordered thoughts and behaviors. The oddest part about this is that I am not a religious person. I'm a spiritual person and do hold a number of personal beliefs, but this is entirely unrelated to the strange things that went through my mind during these most difficult years.

I found that whenever I fasted for long periods of time or went for so many weeks with an extremely low-calorie intake, that I would develop a feeling of euphoria. I felt as if I was light, and free, and *sinless*—almost as if by refusing food I was rejecting all notions of gluttony, and in doing so was somehow purifying my soul of something. It was almost like getting a power kick from this idea that formed inside my head and told me that I was capable of reaching some field of soul immortality, one that was completely untarnished by the 'toxins' of the external world.

Looking back on that now, from where I am in my life at this point, I can't even begin to understand where those thoughts came from. Even I found it bizarre to read through those journals, and it all came from my own head!

However, there was also a far darker side to the actions I took while in the midst of my eating disorder. Ultimately, everything I did ended up not only being a way for me to try and grasp at some control, but also a way for me to deal with the stress of living and my feelings of depression at that time. Hunger made me feel euphoric, binging gave me comfort, and purging felt like an appropriate action of self-punishment for all the things that I hated about myself.

I would like very much to be able to say that all of this is in the past—especially considering just how self-aware I have become of not only my actions but also the consequences of these actions—but it is not. I still go through cycles in which things are bad, as well as times when things are good, and my disordered eating habits still reflect this.

One thing to which I have become more attuned in the last year or so is that these particular thoughts are largely dependent on the other things that are going on in my life. I have found that when I feel at my most comfortable and supported, then these thoughts are less of an issue. This tends to be because I feel propelled to excel in other aspects of my life, and so am less dependent on searching for control and success through unhealthy means.

But old habits die hard, and it isn't always the case that support equals resolution. There have been times when I've been in the most supportive environments imaginable and have still been preoccupied with disordered thoughts, and then there have also been times when I've been in mentally damaging environments, and somehow managed not to slip back into negative behavior patterns.

Sometimes, both love and logic have a tendency to kick me in the ass and point out all of the reasons why recovery is so infinitely better than the suffering I've become accustomed to putting myself through over the years. And due to this, I can go for months not worrying too much about the things that, on other occasions, often try to consume my life. But when bad things swing around again, then I find that I can be very easily triggered into falling back into old, self-destructive routines, and my brain suddenly becomes this foreign enemy that won't let the love or the logic get through anymore.

These days, one thing that I certainly see a lot of in my social circles is the conversation about the difficulties involved when it comes to accessing help for eating disorders, and the truth in this is overwhelming. Personally, I have found it very hard to get any help from doctors, because they seem to run everything through a tick list system. And if you don't fall into a specific category... well, *no help for you!*

In my case, I was not really 'into' seeking help. For a long time, I didn't recognize a problem; and then once I did, I was scared to admit the problem; and then once I admitted the problem, I didn't fall into a nice tick list category. And so, due to this, I managed to convince myself on some level that I actually must have been mistaken in the first place, and that there wasn't really a problem after all.

I found that trying to get professional help was specifically difficult when mixed with the external pressure to do better. Because I became aware of the impact that my eating disorder can have on my physical health, and thus the impact that it can have on the people I care about the most, I wanted to try to do better. I wanted to do better for those I loved. However, the positive progress that can be made purely by the want to be better is then almost undermined by the healthcare system. It somehow manages to turn a good thing into a bad thing.

For example, managing not to partake in certain disordered behaviors for a certain amount of time (even if that amount of time is actually rather short, in the long run) can then disqualify you from a section on the tick list. Regardless of whether or not this positive change is something that can be sustained all on your own, or how easy it is to slip back through the cracks, you magically become ineligible for certain types of support—and when your eating disorder behaviors are cyclical, like mine, getting help can be practically impossible.

So, what I always try to do is just keep in mind during my darkest moments that I am loved, even when I can't feel it. I have to constantly tell myself that I do have people who care about me and want me to do well, even if I can't make myself believe it. For me, the repetition is key.

A huge step for me in regards to trying to do better was learning not to weigh myself, and this was something that I could never have done all on my own. I was obsessed with the scale for a long time and was very specific about the time of day and state of undress I had to be in to even step on. This obsession was so strong that there was no way that I was going to be able to quit cold turkey, and so I am incredibly grateful for the support I received from a family member in being able to do this.

This originally came about by the scale being put out for me on Monday mornings, so that I could weigh myself at the same time every week—but only once a week, as opposed to every single day, as I had been doing previously. There then happened to be an occasion of about two weeks when I did not have access to the scale (which was due to traveling) and after that, I just stopped asking for it. This was primarily because some time had passed and I didn't know if our arrangement was still standing, and—being the awkward person that I can be—I was just too nervous to ask.

However, there is no option in my life for never stepping on the scales again, as my physical health issues mean that I see doctors rather a lot, and they do like to weigh people. Being weighed by the doctor was something that I always feared because it wasn't done *my* way. I couldn't stand the numbers on the scale because they included the weight of my clothing and any food or drink I had consumed that day before being weighed. And despite the fact that the logic of all this was present in my head, it still made me feel awful about myself to see those numbers as higher than the ones I was used to. But I did discover that it didn't have to be like that.

In fact, just before my last MRI, I didn't look at the scale at all, and I really do owe this entirely to the same family member who incited the change in my relationship with the scale in the first place. She came with me on a trip to the doctor on a previous occasion and was the first person to somehow manage to convince me that I didn't have to look at the scale when they weighed me. She even told the nurse not to say it out loud, because she knew that I'd obsess over it if she did.

I didn't realize this at the time, but this was actually one of the most helpful things to happen with my mindset surrounding my preoccupations with food and weight. I mean, it obviously made a positive difference if almost a year later, and 5,000 miles away, I actively chose not to look at the hospital scales. Because she truly made me believe that the number did not define me, and I didn't have to know what it said or let it dictate my actions, as it had done so many times before.

But as far as I have come in certain aspects regarding my turbulent relationship with food, I do think it's important just to point out that I am not yet recovered. As I've mentioned already, I go through periods of time, and countless cycles, in which my brain has not yet accepted that I am enough. Has not yet quite realized that I am a capable and perfectly acceptable specimen of a human being. I have tried for what feels like a long time (and I will continue trying) to reach a state where I am able to embrace the concept of self-love. But in the meantime, I am who I am, and I have the body I have, and it changes as my mental state changes.

The biggest thing I've come to realize, however, is that this does not mean that my body is any less worthy of being what it is. Yes, my body is sick, my mind is sick; and, in my case at least, even once my mind reaches a point at which it is more content, my body will continue to be sick, because (as I have already discussed at some length) my health issues span far beyond just my eating disorder.

A body does not have to be in a recovered state to deserve the recognition that it is valid and acceptable, and to simply be a part of this world. And the brain that comes part and parcel with this body does not require to be whole, or healthy, or perfect to give it justice.

I mean, I still do not like my body. I still do not feel comfortable with it. But it's what I have, a part of what makes up the three-dimensional existence of who I am. It's not my be-all and end-all, it's only the physical form that I hold, and carry around, and what's on show to the rest of the world most of the time.

But it *is* a part of me. It has parts that are squishy, and parts that are pointy, and parts that are speckled and scarred. Perhaps I like some of these things; perhaps I hate some of these things. And perhaps my opinion changes depending on my daily mindset. But despite what my mindset may be—despite what I may be thinking at any particular point in time—my body is mine, and I have to accept it, unconditionally, as it is right now. It will change—of course it will change, *that's life*—and that's okay. Because all it really does is show that I am alive.

Because I *am* alive. And *you* are alive.

You are alive, and you take up space, and that's okay. Your body will change. But it's yours, and it has no impact on who you are, or how good you are, or how worthy you are. You, as a person, are loved, no matter your size. The body is just the form of what is loved. You are not defined by your three-dimensional earthly existence, and those who love you don't even see it. Your body is a reminder that you are here. You are a person, and this is the world, and you have a part in it. You are loved in it. You are *you* in it.

The main thing that I have learned—and believe me when I say that this has been a very recent discovery, and one that I can't really take credit for—is that self-love achieves so much more than self-hatred ever will. And no one should feel the need to do what I did, and keep struggles like this a secret for years from the fear of being judged—of being seen as less than capable, less worthy of support and trust due to a perceived inability to look after yourself—because you are worth so much more than your brain may let you believe.

CHAPTER #5

Caught in the Gray

"I am terrified by this dark thing that sleeps in me; all day I feel its soft, feathery turnings, its malignity."
– Sylvia Plath

Depression is another thing that I have struggled with since adolescence and is something that has really been a tremendous driving force behind a lot of what has taken place in my life, as much as I wish this were not the case. Looking back over not only my journal entries from my younger teenage years but also my fictional works of writing, I could see very clearly just how much of my headspace was enveloped in this melancholic haze.

I think, perhaps, one of the most considerable impacts that this had was on my ability to socialize at my first high school. I mean, it wasn't that I was a social hermit or anything, and I did have friends—in fact, the two closest friends I have to this day are people that I attended that school with—but I never really felt comfortable. There was actually this one bathroom in the Sports department where I would just sit and cry, sometimes, during lunch breaks. This was never due to anyone else being specifically mean to me—I wasn't bullied at school—but rather, was caused by my own mental state.

I spent so much time feeling so disconnected from the world in which I lived, that I had no idea how to mingle with people properly. It was like my brain was not on the same field of thought as many of the people around me, and I just couldn't find any interest in the things that seemed to bring them together. The jovial frivolities that seemed central to how other students would interact with one another simply did not capture my attention. Essentially, I was just too sad, anxious, and confused to find joy in the things that brought others closer.

Something that made this time in my life particularly difficult was the tendency for what I was experiencing to be shrugged off as 'teenage angst.' Now, there are few phrases on this Earth that I hate more than 'teenage angst,' and this is for multiple reasons.

One of these reasons is because teenagers do go through a lot of hormonal changes, which can wreak havoc on the brain, but this doesn't mean that what is being felt is any less valid, even if it is just a developmental 'phase.' It can still hurt; it can still lead to self-destructive behavior. During puberty, the brain literally reboots its entire system, and in this process of change, the prefrontal cortex (the bit that deals with consequences of actions, impulse control, etc.) is the last to be developed. This means that the brain is essentially running off the amygdala (which is pretty much *all* impulse, emotion, and animalistic, instinctive behavior) for a good few years.

I also dislike how the word 'angst' is thrown around in this phrase as if it's meaningless. *Angst—a feeling of dread, anxiety, or anguish.* This is an emotion as valid as happiness or grief. If anything, it's more than that—it's a description given to the feeling of man that free will is both appealing and terrifying. Which is true. It's essentially Existentialism. It has literally intrigued philosophers for thousands of years, and yet is commonly discarded as something of little consequence.

However, the main reason I hate this phrase so much is that I find it to be horrendously undermining. Yes, okay, for some it is a developmental 'phase,' and it can be really difficult at the time, and then pass as the years go by. But this is not true for everyone, and there is a real difference between the rollercoaster ride of teenage hormones and mental illness, which a lot of people seem to casually ignore when the sufferer is of a certain age. By referring to someone's mental illness as 'teenage angst,' you may as well be saying, "You'll get over it." But that's just not the reality for us.

My years of depression have also often been coupled with self-harm. And as with so many things that lie in the fog that is my past, I don't remember when this started, but it has been a part of my life for a long time.

Something I find very interesting about this is that I never self-harmed while I was at boarding school. It was almost as if when I was in that more positive environment, there was a part of my brain that told me I couldn't self-harm because in doing so, I would somehow be tainting the good with the bad. I felt as if I couldn't bring that huge weight of negative energy near the hallowed ground that was my boarding school life. But what's ironic here, though, was that I somehow failed to recognize that my eating disorder was doing that anyway.

However, although I never self-harmed when I was actually living at school, I had no such mental restraints whenever I found myself back in situations that were not so supportive and discovered that I could easily still slip back into bad ways. I guess the major question then becomes concerned with why I felt the need to self-harm in the first place, especially considering that the actions themselves seemed to ebb and flow depending somewhat on external factors (like environment).

Thinking back, the main reason I self-harmed, I suppose, was because it reminded me that I was still alive. There would be times when I would hold my flesh to scolding metal, in some attempts to try and rejoin my mind with the body from which I felt so disconnected—as if I were a welder, who could melt the pieces back together with heat. Other times, I would slice open my skin just to see if I could still feel—if I could still *bleed*—and to prove to myself that I continued to exist. But another reason, one that happened to be a significant factor in why I did most of what I did, was this overwhelming need to punish myself for all of my perceived failings.

My whole life, I have never felt good enough; and yet, I am unsure as to what it is that I'm not good enough for, exactly. I am not someone who has ever been subject to external pressure put on me to live up to a certain standard, and yet I still always felt like I was somehow failing.

I think, perhaps, that the thing I feel like I'm not good enough for is actually just life in general. I have this overwhelming sense of insecurity in my own existence, and my harshest critic has always been myself. I often look at those who are older than me, and people who have lived through things so much harder than I could ever imagine, and I don't understand how they do it—how are they still alive? What is their secret? And why don't I feel capable of doing the same? I once met a woman in her 90s, who commented on my smoking habit and asked me if I wanted to live as long as her, and my automatic response was, "Not really."

There was a point where I knew I'd hit a particularly bad place in regards to my depression because of some of the things I came to notice when studying an online business course. This was due to the fact that, in this course, there would be encouragement in the form of thinking about your 'Weekly Wins' and 'Weekly Goals,' as well as prompts about little acts of self-care you did every day to keep yourself motivated. I realized that things were not good when my 'Weekly Win' became having not killed myself yet, and my 'Weekly Goal' was to survive until the next week. Oh, and my daily act of self-care? That was brushing my teeth, and, to be honest, I often failed to keep up with that.

For as long as I can remember, I've always had this part of

me that keeps professing that everything I do is wrong—the things I say, how I say them, how I connect with other people—and the impact of this tends just to make me want to curl up into a ball and disintegrate. I live with this constant dread of how I come across to people, as I touched upon lightly in the first chapter with regards to my anxiety over people even reading this, and what they might think.

The sentence I often feel could pretty much sum up my entire existence is, "No puedes deletrear decepcionante sin Iona." This translates to, "You cannot spell disappointing without Iona," and only really works in Spanish.

However, one way in which this insecurity affects me the most is when it comes to the people I love. I am the kind of person who wants to pull people closer, especially during those periods when I can't deal with the weight of simply being myself all on my own. But at the same time, I'm absolutely terrified of dragging those I care about the most into the turmoil that goes on inside my head, because the fear of it pushing them away is suffocating.

Within my mind, I am constantly engaged in these internal battles of self-hatred. It's like I have a complete inability to understand why anyone in the world would ever love and care for me, because (as far as my brain is concerned) all I ever do is make everything difficult. And due to these feelings, I just end up hating myself for all the inconveniences I cause, and my general incompetence when it comes to being a person makes me feel that no one else could possibly truly *like* me, forget about *love* me.

One of the main insecurities I have is the idea that the whole world sees me just as I see myself, hates me as much as I hate myself, and there is a part of me that doesn't believe in love or kindness when I find it. A part of me always thinks that the love that I do find from people is either a lie, or something that they get into with me without realizing what that means, or how much they're taking on. And then I just wait for it to all fall apart.

Something I have come to learn, though, is that even having these thoughts in the first place has a tendency to make things worse. In feeling, on some level, that the love and support I experience isn't real—you know, since my head is just waiting for everyone to start hating me as much as I hate myself—it can result in me inadvertently acting odd in certain situations when I'm feeling particularly vulnerable, and so can become sort of like self-sabotage. But the thing about this is that I can't prevent it. I cannot stop these thoughts from permeating around my head, and I am often unaware of any subsequent strange behavior until *after* it has taken place—which, by that point, makes it too late.

These insecurities are also compounded with a strong sense of isolation. Now, when I refer to this isolation, I mean it in a literal sense. Due to the physical limitations that I experience, and sometimes also just certain life circumstances that take place, I often find myself very closed off from the world. There have been multiple occasions when I have found myself stuck indoors, with very limited mental stimuli, and a distinct lack of social interaction.

The biggest issue this has posed for me is that being disconnected from the world in this way means that I end up with far too much time spent alone with my own thoughts, which is never a good thing. When I have this seemingly infinite stretch of time laid out before me, and little to keep my mind occupied, I have a tendency to sit and overthink every detail of my life. During these times, I frequently do this to such an extent that I either get too caught up in all the bad things and repeatedly go over all of my past mistakes, or I become stuck remembering all the good things that have ever happened and feel unable to deal with the fact that they are not the present.

I often find it very difficult to look back at all the amazing times in my life, because these periods of intense overthinking result in me somehow being able to turn the best things in my life into negative things. It's like I have this voice in my head that keeps telling me that these great memories are only in the past, that they don't exist anymore, and that I'll never have them back. It turns into this awful comparison of, "That was then, but this is now… and now really sucks!" And it makes me believe that the happiness is over and will never come again.

Something else about the mixture of isolation with the continually playing broken record of memories is that it makes me compare not only events in my life but also relationships. When I'm alone for such a long period of time, it makes me wonder where all the people have gone. It's like being a kid and walking through a crowded street holding your mom's hand. But then, somewhere along the road, the hand slips from your grasp, and no matter how much you look around you, you can't find her among the bustling group of strangers—and suddenly, you're lost. If I don't have a regular source of contact, then *I* start to feel lost and think that no one loves me anymore.

Rationally, I know that this is not the case, and just because the days feel like years to me when I'm alone doesn't mean that time stops for other people. There are a few people with whom I'm very close and will not get a reply for two or three weeks after sending a text message, and this can be a totally normal occurrence. And when I'm out living life and being a person, then I barely even notice, because I am also someone who is busy doing things. However, when I'm just sitting on my own, not doing anything, and not having anyone around, two or three weeks can feel like a lifetime, and my mind starts to play tricks on me.

For example, one text that I genuinely sent to my best friend during one of these times said, "Being without human interaction for so long now has me questioning if I might actually have died without realizing? I don't even get spam email anymore."

It may sound a little crazy, but when I find myself in these situations, I do go kind of crazy. Without other people to remind me that I still exist, I begin to run all of these worst-case scenarios through my head. Of course, I don't actually fully believe that I may have died without realizing (at least, that hasn't happened yet, anyway), but the lack of communication—or perhaps, sometimes, the *perceived* lack of communication—does lead me to continually question what it was that I did wrong for no one to want me anymore, for that grasp of hands to be loosened. And these particular thoughts really can lead me into a downward spiral of depression.

When I speak about my downward spiral in this context, what I'm referring to is hysteria—real, heaving, mind-blowing hysteria. For me, these episodes are characterized by crying to the point of being unable to breathe, sobbing that wracks my chest and leaves me howling silent screams because I can't get enough air together to do anything other than just sit and hyperventilate. And then, after some time—30 minutes, an hour, maybe two—it all just suddenly stops. It's like someone has flipped a switch, and everything goes numb; mind blanked, body frozen, breath hanging in the still air.

The main thing about these episodes that I find hardest to deal with is the fact that they can appear almost completely out of the blue. Sometimes this is specifically true to form (like when I fall into a bout of hysterics that's connected with seizure activity). Other times it's more to do with something being sparked in my mind that causes me to cry, which in turn can progress into a full-blown attack of hysteria due to the lack of any external reasoning force to bring me out of my head and back to reality. Then, when it does stop, and the numbness rolls in, there is some time where I just don't feel anything anymore. Often, at this stage, I just tend to fall asleep—it is, quite literally, emotional exhaustion.

And these events happen over, and over, and over again. Sometimes there can be months between them, and other times they can be a daily (or, more commonly, *nightly*) occurrence, but they always come back. And it really is, as I just said, absolutely *exhausting*.

Going through bouts like this also has a way of opening up my insecurities. The fact that I find myself so unable to deal with my emotions at certain points in time makes me feel incredibly infantile—and I hate this; I want to *have* a baby, not *be* a baby. But in these moments, I have that same sensation that I experience during my MS relapses, and it's like I'm suddenly a toddler again.

During these periods of isolation, I cry because I'm lonely, and eventually stop because I realize that I'm alone—no one is going to come hold me and make it all okay. And most of the time, *thank fuck for that!* Because I am not comfortable with people seeing me in the state that these episodes leave me in. Many people have seen me cry, but I can count the number of people to see me in hysterics on one hand. Luckily for me, those who have borne witness to these episodes have generally been the 'right' people—family who loved me anyway, and at times, actually did hold me and make it all okay.

But even with them, I still felt embarrassed and ashamed

afterward and wanted nothing more than to apologize for it all, and beg them not to think differently of me. The primary reason for this internal response is, once again, linked to my own sense of insecurity and the fear that other people seeing me in that condition means that they'll just want to leave because it's too difficult to deal with—because *I'm* too difficult to deal with. However, the thing I have to remember is that this response is entirely my own; I cannot read minds, and so it is not possible for me to know what anyone else may be thinking in these moments.

CHAPTER #6

Consumed by the Sin

*"Why did I feel I needed to be punished, to punish myself.
Why do I feel now I should be guilty, unhappy: and feel
guilty if I am not?"*
– Sylvia Plath

When it comes to the state of your physical and mental health, I think something that makes all of it substantially more difficult to deal with is the voice in your head that can make you feel ashamed for all of the perceived failings or inabilities that come as part of this terrain.

In regards to my physical disabilities, I often feel guilty about the fact that I am not always able to be an independent adult on my own and that other people quite frequently have to drop what they're doing and stop or rearrange a bunch of stuff in order to take care of me. As I discussed in Chapter 2, MS relapses mean that, at times, I'm not able to do the most basic of things (like prepare food, walk up stairs, etc.) and so what that results in is other people having to put their day on hold, or change their schedules, to help me with some simple aspects of just being alive. The same goes in relation to my epilepsy, except that this also comes with the added task of ensuring that certain activities are safe for me to do and won't trigger seizures.

There are also times when I try to do the independent things anyway, and end up being unsuccessful or getting hurt. That then makes me feel even guiltier about the fact that someone else has to pick up the pieces from an action that was actually the direct result of me trying to do something that I, perhaps, maybe should not have attempted in the first place.

For instance, if I were in MS relapse, and was feeling guilty over being dependent on someone else for doing all the washing up in the kitchen, then I might try to help by putting away some plates. However, if I'm lacking the strength in my arms to carry things properly, or lack the coordination in my legs to walk steadily, then I may drop the plates or fall over, which then results in smashed plates and possibly minor injuries due to broken shards. This then means that the person on whom I was dependent for doing these things no longer just has the simple task of putting away the dishes, but now has to clear up a bunch of broken plate pieces, and may also have to deal with any cuts I might have sustained.

Situations like this are awful because my intentions are pure, and yet no matter what I do it always seems to be wrong, and the guilt is overwhelming. It's like there is no correct answer or right action that I'm supposed to take—just a bunch of problems with no comfortable solution. All I can do is keep in mind that the responsible and adult thing is to accept the fact that I am not fully functional all the time, and trying anyway is likely to cause more harm than good.

I tend to notice this the most when it comes to my family and the people that I love, because it makes me feel so awful to think that even having me in their lives at all means dealing with this huge amount of intrusive baggage that I bring with me. And it's not only the people I love, but also just people who are unfortunate enough to even be near me at the 'wrong' time in regards to where my health is at—like the people I went to school with or the strangers on the bus from another seizure event that I neglected to mention earlier (I'm sure you can take a guess). But whether talking about family, friends, acquaintances, or complete strangers, I feel like it's not their problem to deal with me, and yet I somehow manage to inadvertently make it their problem every time I'm around anyone else on this Earth.

When it comes to my mental health, the feelings are pretty much the same. The issues that I experience with my mental health, and my subsequent actions and reactions in certain circumstances, carry those same feelings of guilt because I hate the impact it all has on other people.

In my head, it's like I have this constant internal battle between attitudes of, "Remember me, but let me go," and, "Please don't give up on me, I promise I'll do better." The reason for this is that half the time, I just want not to exist anymore and wish I could dissolve into the ether; and the other half of the time, I become overwhelmed by loneliness and the fear that if I can't pull myself together, then everyone I love will leave. But the issue with this is that both of these mindsets make me feel ashamed of being who I am. I end up feeling guilty for the thoughts of wanting to leave because there's something in that which feels very selfish, especially when people have tried to help me, because I imagine it to seem incredibly ungrateful. But I also feel guilty for the thoughts that seem to put other people too much at the center of why I want to try harder, because I fear that's too much pressure to put on them—how long can I really expect people to hang around if my positive changes never seem to stick?

I feel like, in general, we all want to be strong for the people around us. And when we can't be the person we wish we were inside our heads, then it makes us feel guilty for not living up to what we think we should be. This, in turn, feeds the cycle.

This is especially poignant when these feelings manifest as not being able to manage situations or relationships correctly. When I am in a particularly bad slump and act oddly, or can't seem to pull myself together, or simply cannot stop crying, then I find that this also falls on the people around me, even when I don't mean for it to do so. When I feel overwhelmed, I make things weird, and then I feel bad about the fact that I didn't control myself better. Due to this, I often don't reach out to anyone when I'm in a bad place, because I don't want to add to anything else that may be going on in that other person's life.

This feeling of guilt when I do make situations (and, subsequently, relationships) strained, tends to result in me retreating into a shell, which actually makes it all worse because then I end up being awkward when trying to reconnect to the world due to the fact that I believe everything is my fault. My brain tells me over and over again that I'm a burden and only make everything harder than it has to be—that I make good things bad and bad things worse—and then I feel guilty that I can't also be the person to fix those situations.

It's somewhat well-known that no one wants to be around a downer, and so I understand entirely the irritants that I can cause during the times when my brain is stuck in negative places and I can't hide that fact from either my face or my actions. But I do not want to be a downer, and I'm not always! Sometimes I can be a highly entertaining human being. However, I do not have control over these emotions—when they come and go, and to what extent the bad waves hit me—and I hate it. I always feel very guilty whenever I make things awkward or uncomfortable, especially when the situation is caused simply by the fact that I can't deal with being a person.

However, when I happen to be in such a place where I am able to have moments of clarity, I see just how unfair these thoughts of mine are. If I were to remove myself from the situation and view it as a third party, then my thoughts and beliefs would change entirely. In doing this, it enables me to see just how much of what goes on inside my head—and what can occasionally spill out of my head and into my actions—is rooted quite deeply in a strong sense of self-hatred, and is not really true at all.

When I really think about it, it feels unfair to both myself and everyone else to be so stuck in this guilty mindset—because if one of us is guilty, then we're all guilty, right? And it is not up to me to say that. It is not up to anyone to say that. Not even when we're saying it to ourselves.

There are so many other people out there who are in the same position as I (if not worse), so why do I spend so much time feeling awful about myself, but don't judge others for the same perceived failings? I have this tremendous sense of guilt for all the things that I've ruined or people I've inconvenienced when I've had seizures, but I don't look at other people who have epilepsy and think, "Wow, you're such an inconvenience, I do not want to hang out with you." So why do so many of us feel this way about ourselves, regardless of whether we're thinking about physical or mental health? We do not judge others for what they cannot control, and yet we beat ourselves bloody for every minuscule movement that we feel could have gone better. I may feel guilty, but none of us should.

I've always felt like a burden, but never really knew what to do about it. In fact, I didn't even know there was anything I *could* do about it. I've always thought that this was just me, just who I am. I've often felt as though I could be summed up as the embodiment of an oxymoron—simultaneously not enough, and also far too much to deal with.

I have this part of my brain that tells me that I am just inherently not good enough: not good enough for myself, and certainly not good enough for anyone else. There have been times when I've been entirely convinced that all I did was bring problems to other people's lives and that everyone would grow to dislike me, if they didn't already. Even those who loved and cared for me the most—it was as if I was just waiting for them to realize their mistake, and then when they did, they'd walk away.

But what I have come to realize, in these moments of clarity, is that all of these thoughts that worsen the pain within my head and heart are just that—they are *thoughts*, not facts, and I do not have to listen. As I said, I didn't know there was anything that I could do about the way my brain sometimes makes me feel, but *this* is what I can do about it—I can learn not to listen.

However, I do firmly believe that this is easier said than done; you can't just eradicate a lifetime of self-hatred and negative thought patterns by knowing that you shouldn't listen to them anymore, because they still make a lot of noise and simply deciding that you don't want to hear it anymore doesn't mean that you suddenly know how to do that. I don't know how to do that. I'm still learning.

Because that's what this is—it's a learning process, and this learning process can be made a lot smoother when we have the right support.

One thing that I really don't like is when people say, "You

have to do better for yourself, not anyone else," because sometimes we can't. Or at least we can't all start off this way, anyway. This is because when you hate yourself to the point where you do not want to exist, you can't just transition straight into being better for yourself, because you don't feel worthy of anything that entails. And when you're in this mindset of worthlessness, then things such as self-care don't appear to you as self-care, but instead appear as selfishness, and so you can't do it—you don't feel *worthy* of doing it, you don't feel that you *deserve* to do it.

Others can't expect you to just take a step back and magically be brilliant at being a person—you have to learn. It's a process.

Sometimes it is only possible to reach the level of being able to do things for yourself after you've already gotten some practice in by improving yourself with others in mind for a while. Live for the people you love, and you can learn to live for yourself.

Ultimately, we all have our shit, and I think that we all need to be a little more caring and supportive of one another, especially those we love. We can't all be all right all the time. That's just life, and I feel like sometimes people forget that.

When you are the person suffering, you forget that other people have had lows just as bad or even worse than yours, and have done things just as bad or even worse than what you have done. You forget, and all you can do is blame yourself for all of your own failings and perceived inabilities to handle life correctly.

And other people forget, as well. Other people sometimes look at you in your bad place and shake their heads, and seem to have a million ways you should be doing better right at the tip of their tongue. But they often forget that they were once where you are—at some point in their life, they, too, have been in a place where things have gone wrong, or they have done things wrong, or they have felt exactly the same way that you might feel.

But we're all only human. And we all forget.

I have seen a phrase passed around that reads, "A person with x y z [whether those things are physical or mental] is not giving you a hard time, they're having a hard time," but in reality, it's both, which is why we have to work together. Part of being a human being is having an impact on one another—sometimes these are good, sometimes they're bad, and sometimes they are both, but can you imagine what the world would be like if we never had these experiences with other people? My guess is that it would be pretty lonely, and I don't much like the sound of that.

It's often said that the goal in life is not just to survive, but to thrive. However, if all you can do at a certain point in time is survive, then do that, and don't feel any less for it. If all you can do is survive, then that's okay. That's more than okay. Don't let anyone else make you feel like that's not enough. Everything else can wait. And don't feel embarrassed or guilty for seeking help or comfort when you need it. Because, in the end, all any of us can do is try to keep on going, and sometimes that means finding support when you're at your most vulnerable.

But here's the important thing to remember: you are not a problem. And try not to let the pressures of society make you feel inadequate. You are wonderful the way you are, flaws and all. That's what makes us who we are. There's nothing wrong with breaking; you can fill the cracks with gold.

CHAPTER #7

Hope of Morning

"I want to talk to everybody as deeply as I can. I want to be able to sleep in an open field, to travel west, to walk freely at night."
– Sylvia Plath

Life is a complex and confusing thing to be a part of, and we're all thrown into it without so much as an instruction manual to tell us what the hell it is we're actually supposed to be doing. It's essentially a lot of guesswork and seeing where different circumstances and choices happen to take us, what consequences arise from our actions, and what bonds and memories we create along the way.

Although my brain and body have a way of making life incredibly difficult to deal with at times, what I always try to do is keep certain things in mind, which enable me to hope for a better future. There may be days when being a human is too much for me to handle, but I have to remember that these days will end, and then the next day will come, and I can try again.

The number one thing that keeps me going when I'm feeling

at my worst is remembering that I am loved. As I have previously mentioned, I don't always feel this, and sometimes I manage to turn the good into bad, but calling upon pleasant memories from the past is important because it reminds me that happiness is possible. And yes, this does sometimes also require fighting down the bad thoughts that do, occasionally, try to infect these good memories. But I am able to fight them down, because who is to say that the positive things do not exist anymore and are not coming back? There is no evidence of that. It's just the dark side of my mind playing tricks on me, and (as I said before) I do not have to listen.

I know that I am loved because I have a fantastic family. Even though they are pretty spread out, and large, and really quite complicated, and can be challenging to get in touch with, they do still exist. They do still exist, and they are still there for me—we are there for one another—despite the fact that, sometimes, I forget. And I know this because whenever I see them or call them, then everything suddenly seems better, the world suddenly makes a little more sense, and I'm reminded why I carry on every day. These reminders are important. They keep me going.

I am also lucky enough to have a few really close friends who understand completely the things that I experience in regards to my physical and mental health, and who have likewise had similar experiences or go through similar cycles. What we do is rally together and fight side by side—each in our own way, dealing with our own demons—with the hopes that, one day, we will meet calmer shores. In doing this together, and in supporting one another, we also act as our own reminders that we are not alone.

Just to reiterate something I've already gone over, sometimes we can't be better for ourselves, but we can try for those we love. This is important for me because I am held together quite strongly by the desire to be better for the people I care about the most. Even when I can't be better for me, I can for them.

Whenever I find myself in certain situations with those I love, or when I am even just sparked by a conversation or some sort of interaction with them, my maternal instinct kicks in. Even when it isn't something that can be observed explicitly by my mannerisms or outward actions, there is still a switch in my brain that gets flipped, and my mindset can change in an instant to do anything for the person that I care about, anything at all. When this change occurs, my number one priority becomes protecting them from harm, and that includes the scary side of my mind. A large contributor to the guilt I discussed in the previous chapter is the want to protect those I love from the negativity and self-destruction that lies within my brain, and the feeling of letting them down when I'm unsuccessful in doing this.

However, despite the guilt I have expressed in connection with this way of doing things, being better for others in your life is not a bad thing. That's what happens with the people we love; we try to be the best we can possibly be for them. And, often, they do the same for us. They highlight the good in us, bring the positive attributes to the surface, express the things about us that are the most loveable, and encourage us to be the best versions of ourselves that we can be. My family taught me that, and they led by example.

This is how we grow as people; this is how we learn through love. Be strong for the people you love, and you learn how to be strong for yourself. This is what I do, and it's what I will continue to do. And, maybe one day, I'll finally be able to be better for myself independently of those I love—all the while ensuring that this stronger version of me will be able to hold them up when they feel like crumbling, and carry them just like they've carried me.

One thing I hear all the time in the freelance world is the importance of remembering your 'why.' In business, this is important because it means reminding yourself of all the reasons why you are pursuing a certain career path—it means looking at all the positive outcomes and goals that you have in mind for your business, and what it may enable you to do in your life. This is designed so that you can look back at those reasons whenever things become difficult, and it reminds you *why* you're taking certain classes, or making certain decisions, and what you're working toward. It's motivating. It's what keeps you going when the going gets tough.

This is also something I find to be incredibly helpful when it comes to navigating my life, especially in regards to my health. I find that the same principle applies when it comes to finding the reasons behind doing anything. Like living. When my physical health is at rock bottom, and my mental health is through the floor, and I'm feeling particularly suicidal, *why* do I keep going? For me, my 'why' is my people—it's my family and my future, it's the baby that doesn't exist yet and the life that only lives as a hope inside my head.

The 'why' is important because it encourages me to continue taking steps toward trying to make things better, toward bringing these hopes and dreams out of my head and into the real world. It makes me want to take charge of my future and usher plans to come to fruition; the 'why' tells me the reason I am fighting every single day.

Although I didn't know it at the time, I have actually had this sort of thought process (at least to some degree) since I was a teenager, and what made me realize this was looking at the tattoo I got at 16. Across my left foot, I have ink that reads, "En la guerra no hay sustituto para la victoria" (which means, "In war, there is no substitute for victory," for all you non-Spanish speakers out there) and this acts as a permanent reminder of why I can't stop fighting. Sometimes I forget this—I mean, tattoos just become part of your body, and you sort of stop paying much attention after a while—but I do still believe in what it says, and being able to stop what I'm doing and just stare at the words written on my foot can actually be quite helpful sometimes. A lot of people roll their eyes at 'inspirational quotation' tattoos, but they can be a good thing, I swear.

I am especially influenced by the positive things that can be taken from a good quotation because I am a lover of literature and all things related to writing. Due to this, I find writing to be a very cathartic exercise. I am a person who loves words—I love reading them, I love writing them, and I love to analyze them. Writing has been a part of my soul for as long as I can remember, and I can always find some aspect of the written word to analyze and think about.

As I grew up, the potentially dynamic force that words held grew upon me. I have always been fascinated by what can be exposed through writing—how it can focus on the deepest recesses of the brain in an individual, exploring the events and emotions that make us human. It amazes me that through the act of writing (both fiction and non-fiction experience-based projects, like this one) I have, at times, been able to gain a fresh insight into myself as a human being.

As I said, writing is something that's therapeutic for me, as well as for many others, and I would certainly encourage it as a way to work through emotional stress and trauma. The primary thing I've noted as helpful to me in this exercise has been the ability that writing has given me to put down in words those emotions that run rampant throughout my head. Often, when I am asked questions about the impact that my physical or mental health has on my life, and the things that I am feeling, I cannot verbalize it. I find myself at a loss for words, but only when the words are supposed to be coming straight from my head and out of my mouth.

But given the freedom of the written word, and paper, and time, then I can process everything, and my thoughts magically form into something real and begin to make more sense. Sometimes this results in poetry, other times in prose... and this time, in a non-fiction book that appears to be about my life.

Not everyone is big on writing, but there are lots of other methods of healing through creativity. I've seen and heard some beautiful, haunting, and thought-provoking pieces of art and music, which also stem from the same strand of creative expression as writing. Creative therapy really is an amazing outlet when trying to survive, and I strongly recommend it to anyone who is struggling.

Keeping all of these positive, motivating, and constructive practices in mind has become a vital part of my daily routine because, in doing this, I am able to build up the picture in my head of what I want for my future and how to get there. I have all of these hopes and dreams for my life, and I have to actively summon them as scenarios in my brain so that I know what I'm working toward, and can keep aiming for something.

I know what I want for my future; I am a huge fan of making plans and have planned out pretty much my entire life. Upon hearing this, a lot of people tend to laugh or shake their heads, or just plain tell me how naïve I am for thinking that I can plan these things. But they are wrong. I'm not naïve; I know perfectly well that plans and reality are tremendously different things. And as someone who lives with health issues that can literally appear overnight, I am actually acutely aware of the fact that there are a million varietals that can change everything in an instant. But I cannot live blindly, I have to have a plan, and I know very well that this plan will adapt and change as my life changes. But the plan still has to be there.

So, one of the main parts of this plan is my career. This has certainly taken some turns over the years (as most people's career plans do), but after seriously considering a number of other options—including military service, before I was diagnosed with MS (which people find hilarious, given that I then went on to become a pacifist)—I have happily settled on teaching. I want to be a teacher.

The reasons for this are really quite simple. When I moved to boarding school, I used it as a way to try and reinvent myself in a new place, and leave the baggage of my past behind me. To some extent, this actually worked. As I've said before, I really enjoyed boarding life, and found so many good things in those years, which, ultimately, played a considerable role in shaping the person I am today. And a lot of this was due to having fabulous teachers, and a great school environment that enabled me to flourish.

Now I want to help young people discover new and wonderful things, and inspire fresh minds to think and explore the world around them. I want to be able to give back to younger generations the type of support and encouragement that I received when I was at school. I want to be able to nurture enthusiasm and drive in students, so that they, too, can go out into the world and thrive on what makes them happy—like what English literature and my love of language has done for me.

A lot of what I do to try and keep my physical and mental health in check is also because I want to be a mom in the future. I want to have a baby, and be able to support my child and provide all the care and love they need and deserve. And I refuse to let my seemingly infinite list of inabilities get in the way of that.

I want to get my shit together so that when I have kids, I can be a good mom, and protect my babies. Yes, there are troubles I have that will never leave me, but I will do all in my power to ensure that they are not my kids' problem. My physical and mental health issues are not something that will ever be a secret (I mean, this is literally a whole book about them) but I never want those troubles to become the responsibility of my children. That is one of the primary reasons why I work to better myself as much as I can now, at this age, years before I plan even to start *considering* getting pregnant. Because once I do bring life into this world, I want—*I need*—to be able to do it in a way that holds the best interests of my future child at heart.

In my personal case—as a gay woman who chooses the option of whether and when to try and get pregnant—I can eliminate the possibility of bringing a child into an unstable environment, and I will do everything in my power to ensure that I reach a stage in my life at which I am able to do this successfully, and make a decent life for the little family I want to create.

I also want to see more of the world. I want to be able to explore new places on this Earth and find somewhere I can finally call home. I want to be able to have a house in a good area, where I can bring up my future baby and be happy, and feel a sense of belonging. I want to find somewhere I can harbor, and just breathe. And I am not afraid of working hard to get there.

In this act of constant drowning, I must keep swimming to stay afloat. For me, this mainly involves working on my physical and mental health so that I can keep my head above water long enough to achieve what's required to realize my goals—even if this means I have to fake it 'til I make it for a while. As my foot proudly proclaims, "In war, there is no substitute for victory," and when you're battling strong currents, you cannot allow yourself to go under.

Something that I have come to realize is that being in life for the long run can actually make things easier. As much as I often want it all just to stop, I think over where I used to be, and where I am now. I think about how far I've come, and try to remember all of the good things I would never have experienced had I chosen to quit all those times I wanted to before.

Because that's the thing about going under—it doesn't actually solve any of the bad, it just guarantees that there will be no more future in which to search for the good. It's very difficult to conceptualize the idea of a better future situation when comparing it with a shitty past or turbulent present, and there are no promises that these ideals will ever take place. But there's a far higher chance of realizing this potential when you stick around than if you cut and run.

If you have an awful year and give in to the waves of the world, then you just have an awful year, and that's the end. But if you have ten years and one of them is awful, or even if two or three of them are awful, then you always have the possibility of looking back at that on year ten and thinking, "Wow, wasn't year two a really bad time? And how about year four, wasn't that crap? But here we are, at year ten, and all is well, and there have been eight years of good." But then again, maybe that's just the optimist in me who is able to see it that way. She doesn't come out very often, and so her arguments tend not to be very developed. To be perfectly honest, I'm not even sure how much sense that makes outside my own head, but it works for me when I need it to.

I'm not very skilled at being positive. But I try, every day, because I need to make things better. And when you're an adult, and your people are scattered all over the world, there's no one else to make the things better for you. So, I try to be positive when I can, because I have to, and I'm encouraged to try and keep myself together. Because no one else is going to do it for me.

I frequently think of all the good that has taken place, and how it does actually exist (even though I forget) and how I can go about trying to make it come around again. I also think about all the bad stuff, and I try to learn something from it so that I can deal with things better in the future and not continuously repeat the same mistakes.

When it comes down to it, we can all sit and reminisce about the past—all the bad things that have happened, all the good that's gone or has somehow been misplaced—but, at the end of the day, all any of us can do is try our best to work toward the future, toward life, toward living. No amount of guilt can change what's already taken place, and carrying it around just makes it so much harder to gain any progress toward what we want tomorrow to bring.

Just try to keep in mind, no matter how many storms might come your way or how strong the maelstrom's pull may be, you are not alone in this act of constant drowning. We must hold onto the hope that, someday, we will find ourselves in calmer waters—we just have to remember how to breathe. Do not worry about the time it could take to achieve something like this; as long as you keep swimming, the time will pass anyway. Just do the best you can each day. Sometimes your best mightn't be very good—that's okay, just keep going.

You *are* enough.

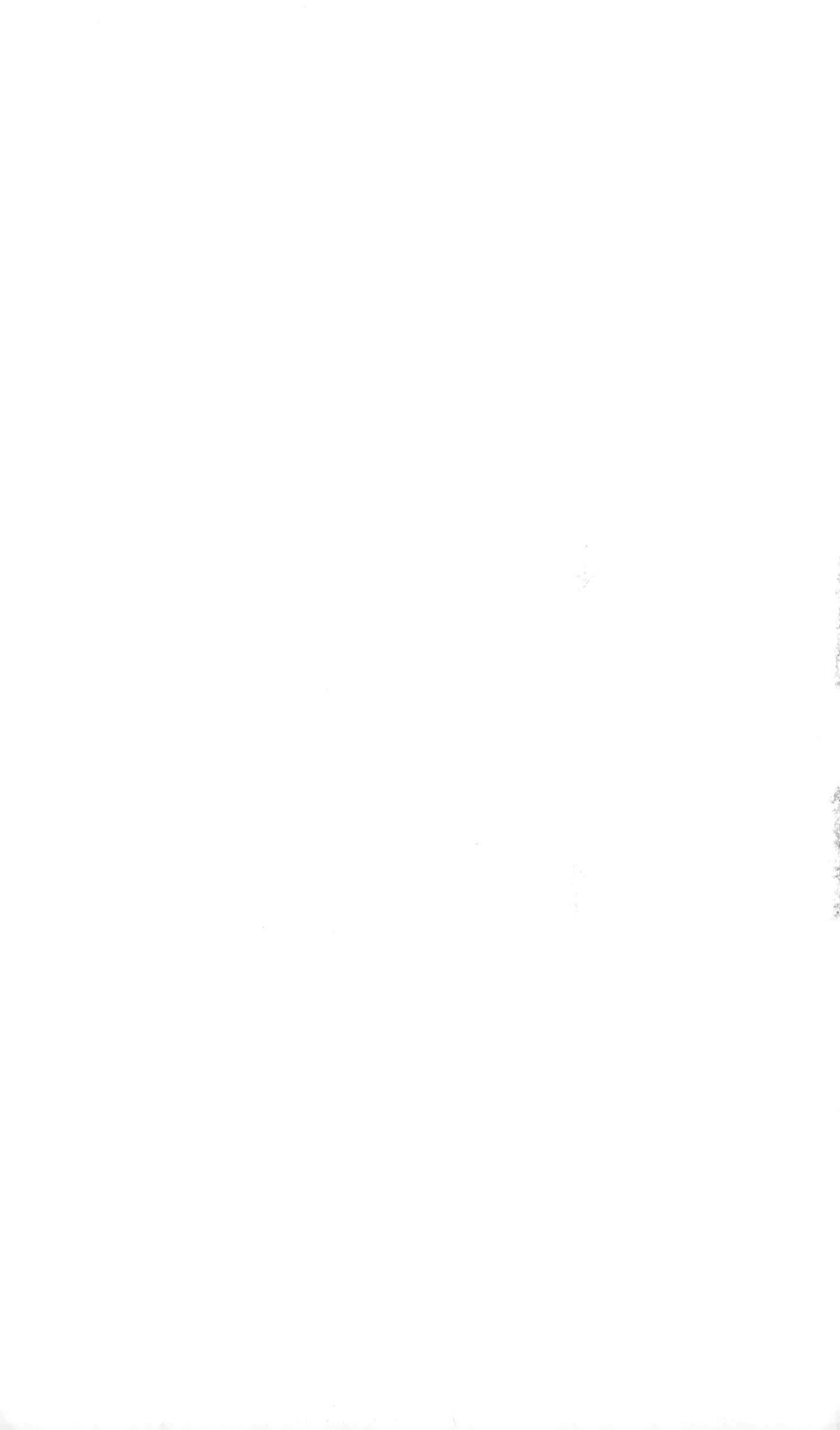

Printed in Great Britain
by Amazon

87007598R00052